TYPE 2 DIABETES FOR BEGINNERS:

25 Steps to Take After Diagnosis, How to Prevent Complications, Nurture Blood Sugar Naturally, & 100 + Diabetic Food List That'll Help You Manage & Stay in Control

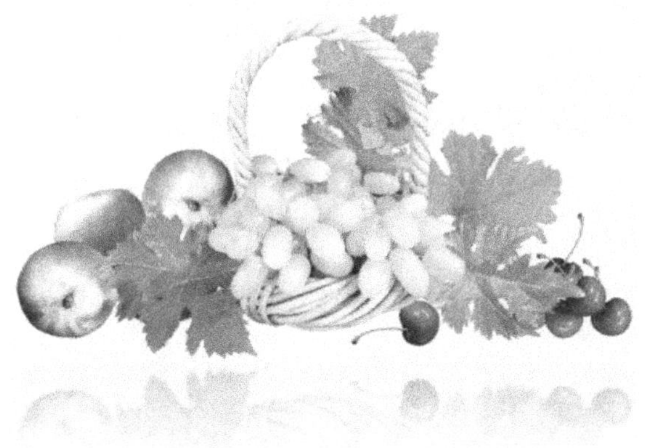

Allison D. Dixon

Copyright © 2024 Allison D. Dixon

No part of this book may be reproduced or transmitted in any form without the prior written permission of the copyright owner.

Disclaimer:

This book is for informational purposes only. The author and publisher are not liable for any damages or losses resulting from the use of the information.

Any resemblance to actual persons or events is purely coincidental.

TABLE OF CONTENTS

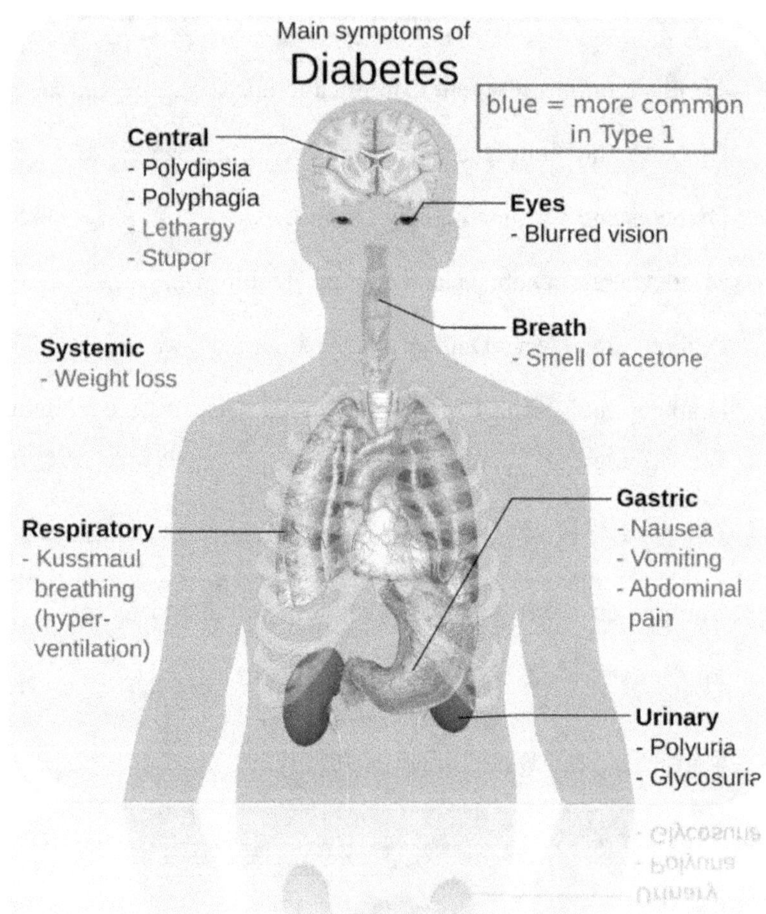

Main symptoms of
Diabetes
blue = more common in Type 1
Central
- Polydipsia
- Polyphagia
- Lethargy
- Stupor
Eyes
- Blurred vision
Breath
- Smell of acetone
Systemic
- Weight loss
Gastric
- Nausea
- Vomiting
- Abdominal pain
Respiratory
- Kussmaul breathing (hyper-ventilation)
Urinary
- Polyuria
- Glycosuria

INTRODUCTION

Welcome to the journey of flourishing with type 2 diabetes. If you're reading this, you could be at the same crossroads that someone close to me once was at: the moment she was diagnosed with diabetes. Let me tell you a secret: you are not alone, and this book is more than simply a manual; it is a buddy who has scen thc route and wishes to illuminate it for you.

Consider this: a fixed moment in time when the words "You have type 2 diabetes" reverberate through your thoughts. It's a tornado of feelings, including astonishment, perplexity, and maybe terror. My mom has been there. But, among this maelstrom, something lovely is waiting to be discovered: the ability to flourish with diabetes.

This handbook is a compilation of my experiences while taking care of my mom and the knowledge of individuals who've turned their diagnosis into a road map for living well. So, take a cup of tea, find a comfortable spot, and let's go on a trip that goes beyond the pages of a book - a journey to reclaim control of your health.

In these chapters, we are investigating life rather than simply diabetes. After receiving your diagnosis, there are 25 critical measures you can do to take charge of your health. When it comes to what's on your plate, this book includes a list of over 100 meals that may help you on your path.

This is not about constraints; it is about empowering. In this book, we'll look at natural methods to maintain your blood sugar, how to recognize issues and avoid complications, and why early treatment is your superhero cape.

However, this book is more than simply facts and data; it is about stories, namely your own. Frequently Asked Questions become answered signposts, transforming uncertainty into clarity. As you read these pages, remember that information is more than simply power; it is your ally, confidant, and co-pilot on this adventure.

So, here's to you: perseverance, prospering, and establishing a life beyond the limits of diabetes. Welcome to an empowering community where your experience is not just understood, but celebrated. This is more than a guide; it is a promise: life with diabetes is about flourishing rather than simply surviving. Cheers to the adventure ahead!

CHAPTER 1

Understanding Diabetes

Diabetes is a chronic (long-term) health disease that alters how your body converts food into energy. The majority of the food we consume is broken down into sugar (glucose) and released into your circulation. When your blood sugar rises, your pancreas releases insulin. Insulin is a key that allows blood sugar to enter the cells of the body and be used for energy.

It occurs when your body either does not produce enough insulin or cannot utilize it as well as it should. When there is not enough insulin or cells cease reacting to insulin, too much blood sugar accumulates in the circulation. Over time, this may lead to major health issues such as heart disease, eyesight loss, and renal disease.

Diabetes affects around 38 million persons in the United States, with one in every five unaware of their condition.

Among these number of Americans living with diabetes, 90-95% have type 2 diabetes.

It was always assumed to be an illness that only affected people over the age of 45, but it now affects children, teenagers, and young adults.

Types of Diabetes

There are three forms of diabetes: type 1, type 2, and gestational diabetes (diabetes during pregnancy).

Type I Diabetes

Type 1 diabetes occurs when your immune system attacks the insulin-producing cells in your pancreas. It can affect anyone; however, it is more prevalent among people under the age of 30. The game plan here includes food planning, keeping track of things, staying active, and incorporating insulin.

Type 2 Diabetes

Now for the star of the show: type 2 diabetes. This one is a little complicated; it kicks in when your body's cells become resistant to insulin. Your pancreas first strives to keep up, but it eventually tires, much like a marathon runner slows down.

Treatments? Meal planning, monitoring, exercise, and, in many cases, medication.

Gestational   Diabetes

Gestational diabetes may occur in pregnant women who have never had diabetes. If you have gestational diabetes, your baby may be at an increased risk of health complications. Gestational diabetes often resolves once your baby is delivered. However, it raises the chance of developing type 2 diabetes later in life. Your infant is more likely to become obese as a youngster or adolescent and acquire type 2 diabetes later in life.

Prediabetes affects around 98 million persons in

the US, accounting for over one-third of the population. More than eight out of 10 of them are unaware they have it. Prediabetes is characterized by elevated blood sugar levels that are greater than usual but not high enough to be diagnosed as type 2.

Prediabetes increases the chance of developing type 2 diabetes, heart disease, and stroke. Fortunately, if you have prediabetes, the good news is that a CDC-approved lifestyle modification program may assist you in taking healthy measures to reverse the condition.

Causes and Risk Factors

Type 2 diabetes is like a puzzle with both genetic and environmental components. If you are over 40, have diabetes in your family, or have African, Arab, Asian, Hispanic, Indigenous, Latino, Pacific Islander, or South Asian ancestry, you may be at a higher risk. Of course, additional weight around the middle, a lack of physical activity, and a few other things can all play a role.

Symptoms

Now, type 2 diabetes does not usually throw out smoke signals, especially if symptoms appear gradually. Some people only get the message when they are coping with other health conditions, such as heart problems or blurred vision. Look for signs such as extreme thirst, frequent toilet visits, or unexpected weight fluctuations. Feeling fatigued, battling with slow-healing cuts, or experiencing tingling in your extremities? These could be red signs.

If you are newly diagnosed, it's okay to feel overwhelmed at first. Contact your healthcare team and enlist the help of family and friends, as diabetes management is a collaborative effort. You've also got this book to aid you in surviving your type 2 diabetes diagnosis.

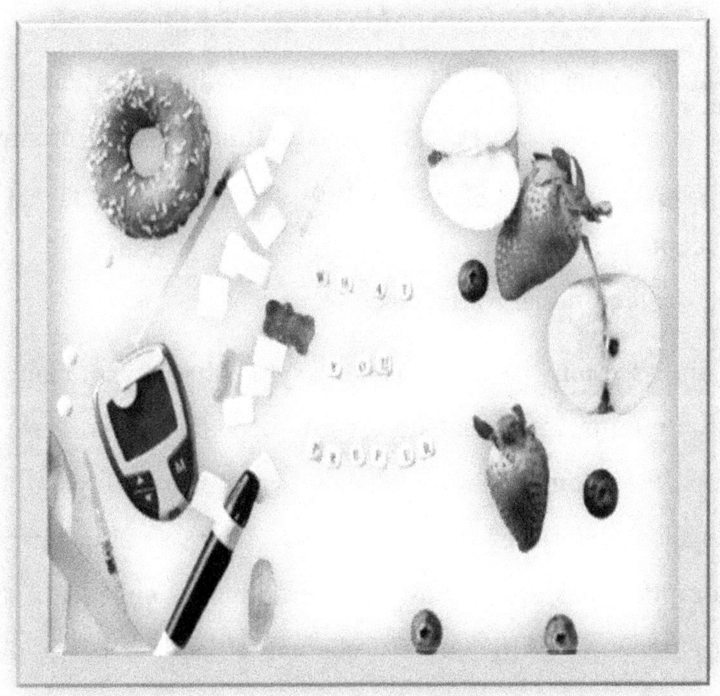

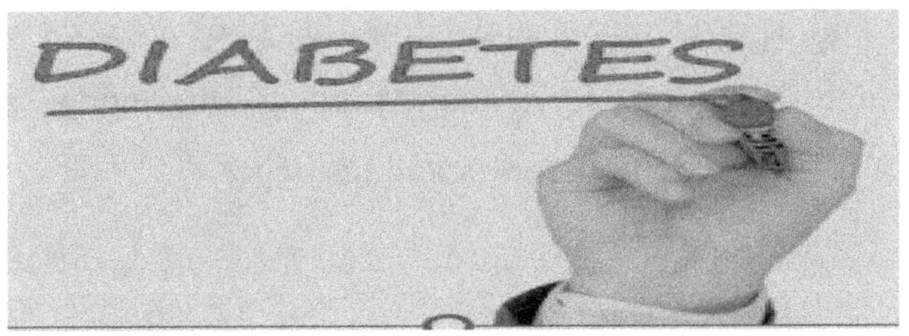

CHAPTER 2

First 25 Steps to Take When Diagnosed with Diabetes

Starting your life with a new diabetes diagnosis can be a very emotional event. It's a voyage filled with uncertainty, changes, and a wide spectrum of emotions, from shock to acceptance. It's critical to recognize that you are not alone on this emotional rollercoaster.

This section serves as a sympathetic companion, highlighting 25 crucial steps for understanding the maze of data that comes with a diabetes diagnosis. Beyond the physical intricacy, these steps address the mental complications, such as the emotional upheaval, the frightening "Why me?" concerns, and the gradual acceptance of the new reality.

So, take a deep breath and allow this book to walk you through the process of understanding, managing, and enjoying a life of more power and resilience.

First Step to Take

Recognize and comprehend the emotions associated with a diabetes diagnosis

Coming to terms with a diabetes diagnosis is acknowledging and understanding the full range of emotions that frequently accompany such news. It's acceptable to feel a variety of emotions, from shock and relief to rage or sorrow. Take the time to study these emotions, allowing yourself to digest and embrace them as necessary parts of your personal path.

For example, knowing your present health status may alleviate the shock of the diagnosis. At the same time, you may grow annoyed with either the situation or yourself. Understanding these emotions is critical to navigating the complexity of diabetes care.

Consider this journey to be a personal story in which each emotion plays a unique role. Accepting and confronting these feelings demonstrates resilience, not weakness. Recognizing and confronting your emotions is a proactive step toward emotional well-being in your diabetes journey.

Second

Dispel the myths

When it comes to diabetes, it's critical to actively research and distinguish between myth and fact. One common misconception is that having diabetes means your life is limited. However, by dispelling such illusions, you give yourself the freedom to live a full and active life.

Consider the belief that diabetics are unable to enjoy sweets. In truth, moderation and intentional choices enable a healthy diet with occasional indulgences. Realizing this may help you overcome restricted beliefs and have a healthier connection with food.

Another common myth is that exercise is unhealthy for diabetes. In truth, frequent physical activity is both safe and healthy. Understanding this allows you to create an activity regimen that is suited to your specific demands and supports general health.

Actively confronting these misconceptions sets the groundwork for a paradigm shift. For example, rather than focusing on perceived restrictions, consider the opportunity for positive lifestyle adjustments.

This myth-busting technique provides correct facts, helping you to adopt a mindset conducive to good diabetes care.

Third

Accept the Reality: Recognize that diabetes will not go away.

Accepting the reality of diabetes is a critical step toward good self-management. Recognize that diabetes is a part of your life, and instead of fighting it, face any challenges that may come. Accepting this truth necessitates implementing the required lifestyle modifications to maintain excellent health.

Consider eating a well-balanced diet, engaging in regular exercise, and monitoring your blood sugar levels. Accepting diabetes as a lifetime condition allows you to take precautions for your long-term health.

Furthermore, diabetes does not change your identity. While it necessitates changes, it does not decrease your value or abilities. Accepting this reality with resilience will enable you to overcome obstacles and continue to live a full, true life.

Fourth

Evaluate Your Health Insurance

Take the time to thoroughly review your health insurance plan, with an emphasis on diabetes-related coverage.

Ensure that your plan covers the medications and supplies required for efficient diabetic care. Pay close attention to details including as premiums, deductibles, and copayments to gain a complete grasp of your financial obligations.

Inquire about coverage for Diabetes Self-control Education and Support (DSMES), as these programs are critical in improving your knowledge and abilities for diabetes management. Being aware of your health plan allows you to get the resources and support you need, which improves your overall well-being.

Fifth Step to Take

Sugar Spy

Keep tabs on that glucose – it's sweet, but too much can be tricky! Make monitoring your blood sugar a high priority in your diabetes treatment plan. Check your blood sugar levels on a regular basis and maintain accurate records to spot patterns and trends over time.

This useful information serves as the foundation for modifying your management plan, allowing you to make more informed decisions regarding your diabetes treatment.

Consistent monitoring reveals how many factors, such as nutrition, activity, and medication, affect your blood sugar levels. Being proactive in monitoring allows you to better adapt to changes and keep optimal control over your diabetic medication.

Sixth

Follow ADA Diabetes Plate Method

To plan your meals, use the American Diabetes Association's (ADA) Diabetes Plate Method.

The American diabetic Association's (ADA) Diabetes Plate Method is a useful approach to diabetic meal planning. Consider your plate to be a canvas, with three sections: 50% non-starchy veggies, 25% protein, and 25% carbs. This basic method improves portion management and makes it easy to manage your nutritional options.

Consider a supper dish packed with colorful veggies like lush greens or vibrant bell peppers, as well as a lean protein source like grilled chicken or fish.

The remaining 1/4 of the plate can be allocated for healthy grains or other healthful carbs. Visually organizing your meals enhances nutritional balance while also aiding in blood sugar control.

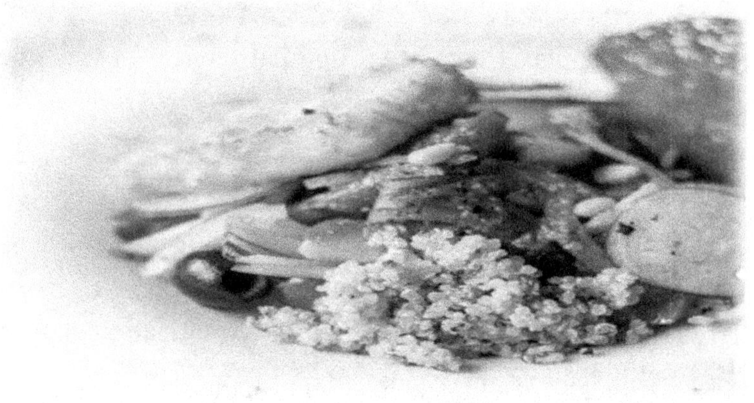

This method not only gives a clear framework for meal planning, but it also promotes a varied and balanced diet. Experiment with different combinations to see what works best for you, and make sure that each plate contains a well-balanced, diabetes-friendly mix of nutrients.

Seventh

Choose Complex Carb

Rather than fully avoiding carbohydrates, make informed choices by choosing complex carbohydrates.

Consume whole grains, legumes, nuts, and a wide range of fresh fruits and vegetables. Consult a trained nutritionist to determine the appropriate amount of carbohydrates for your needs.

Consider this nutritious breakfast option: steel-cut oats topped with a handful of mixed berries and sliced almonds.

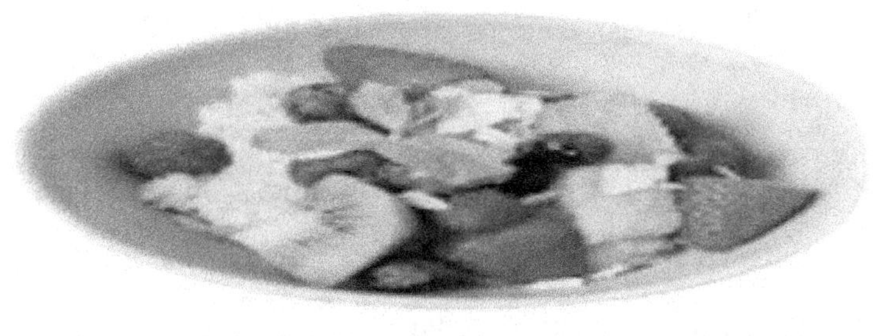

This option not only gives a delicious and nutritious start to your day, but it also contains complex carbs, which aid in the constant release of energy. Incorporating a variety of colorful veggies and legumes into your meals gives a wide range of nutrients while also effectively controlling your blood sugar levels.

Working with a trained nutritionist provides a personal touch to your diet plan. They can evaluate your specific needs, taking into account factors such as exercise level, medication, and particular allergies to foods. This collaborative method adjusts your carbohydrate consumption to maintain stable blood sugar levels, supporting general well-being during your diabetes treatment journey.

Eighth

Be cautious of your beverage selection.

Making conscious judgments about your beverage consumption can help you manage diabetes. Reduce your sugar intake by avoiding sugary beverages and instead choosing healthier options.

Prioritize hydrating fluids like water, sparkling water, unsweetened coffee or tea, and other low-calorie beverages.

Consider the effects of replacing sugary sodas with water or sparkling water in your everyday routine. Making this simple change not only reduces your overall sugar intake, but also helps to improve blood sugar control. Furthermore, introducing unsweetened tea or coffee into your beverage options provides a delicious and savory alternative that does not add excessive calories or have a negative impact on blood sugar.

Being conscious of your beverage choices allows you to stay hydrated while supporting your diabetes management goals. This tiny change can have a positive influence on overall well-being, demonstrating how intelligent drink choices contribute to a healthier lifestyle.

Nineth

Understand how carbs affect blood sugar level

Identify carb-rich foods and pay attention to portion sizes.

Developing a thorough understanding of how carbohydrates affect blood sugar levels is an essential component of successful diabetic control.

Recognize carbohydrate-containing foods and limit portion amounts to maintain optimal blood glucose management.

Distinguish between different types of carbs, focusing on fiber-rich sources in your diet. Vegetables, whole grains, fruits, and legumes are wonderful choices since they provide critical nutrients and promote general health. Fiber-rich carbohydrates are believed to have a slower effect on blood sugar, resulting in more stable and controlled levels.

For example, a well-balanced meal that includes nutritious grains like brown rice or quinoa, as well as a range of colorful vegetables and a moderate quantity of lean protein, demonstrates a carb-conscious diet. This not only improves blood sugar control but also increases nutrient intake, emphasizing the necessity of choosing smart carbohydrate choices in your regular meals.

Tenth Step to Take

Flavor Without Sugar

Instead of using sugar, season your meals using herbs and spices.

Making your meals a joyful experience while sticking to a diabetes-friendly diet requires the creative use of herbs and spices. Instead of relying on sugar for taste, try a variety of aromatic ingredients like cinnamon, garlic, turmeric, and herbs.

For example, a savory stir-fry with a variety of colorful veggies seasoned with garlic, ginger, and a sprinkle of turmeric not only adds depth to the dish but also contains anti-inflammatory effects. This gourmet approach to cooking ensures that your meals are entertaining and satisfying without sacrificing health.

Incorporating herbs and spices creatively not only improves the taste of your meals, but also exposes you to a wide range of nutrients and potential health advantages.

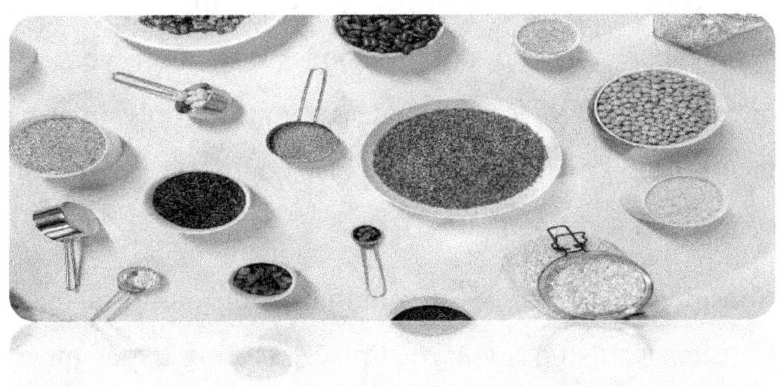

This displays a determined effort to prioritize flavor while maintaining your commitment to efficiently regulating blood sugar levels.

Eleventh

Embrace Mindful Eating

Elevating your dining experience to a mindful practice entails consciously focusing on your relationship with food. Begin by listening to your body's messages and discriminating between actual hunger and other emotional cues.

Allow yourself to enjoy each bite, using your senses to thoroughly absorb the textures and flavors.

To create a mindful dining environment, remove distractions such as smartphones, turn off the TV, and focus your attention on the food in front of you. By intentionally enjoying your meals, you not only improve the sensory experience but also cultivate a healthy connection with food.

Consider this example of mindful eating during a meal. Consider enjoying a colorful salad, savoring the crispness of fresh vegetables, the juiciness of ripe tomatoes, and the perfume of a delicious dressing. Savoring each bite not only promotes a pleasurable dining experience, but also helps to maintain appropriate blood glucose levels.

Incorporating mindfulness into your daily meals can be a transformative experience, allowing you to make deliberate decisions that benefit your overall well-being, including blood glucose management.

Twelfth

Shed a few pounds if overweight

If you're overweight, start with tiny actions to lose a few pounds.

Beginning your journey to a healthier weight

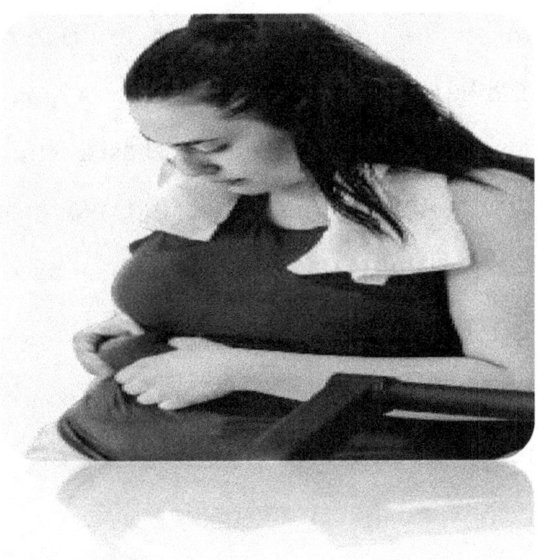

entail taking little steps, with an emphasis on balanced nutrition and increased physical activity.

Consider making minor modifications to your everyday routine, such as choosing nutrient-dense foods and finding fun activities to be more active.

For example, start by adding more fruits, veggies, and whole grains to your meals while progressively reducing portion sizes. This can help to create a well-rounded diet that benefits your overall health. In addition, look into physical activities that make you happy, such as taking a daily walk, cycling, or participating in leisure sports.

Imagine going for a 20-minute brisk walk in the morning and having a colorful salad at lunch. By making these little modifications on a regular basis, you not only help with weight control but also improve insulin sensitivity and blood sugar levels.

By concentrating on attainable goals and rewarding accomplishments along the way, you can cultivate a long-term strategy to weight control that benefits both your health and diabetes care.

Thirteenth

Maintain a steady sleeping routine

Quality sleep has a significant impact on diabetes care. Strive for a consistent sleep routine, averaging 7-8 hours of refreshing sleep per night.

This dedication to adequate and restful sleep is critical for balancing hunger and desires, which influences good blood sugar regulation.

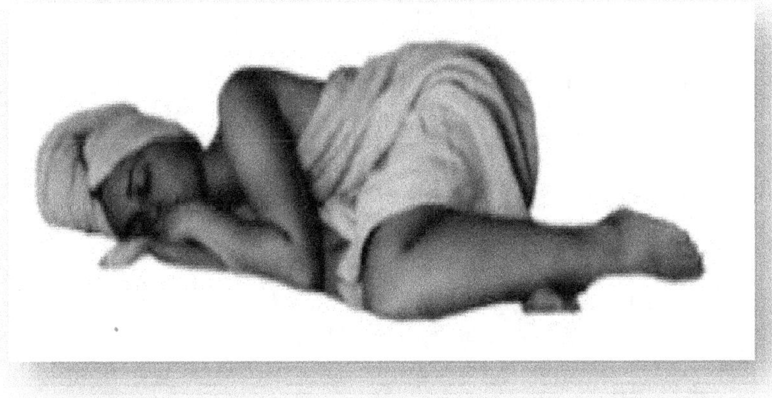

Consider creating a nightly routine to inform your body that it's time to relax. This could include reading, moderate stretches, or practicing relaxation techniques. By creating a suitable sleep environment, such as keeping your bedroom chilly and limiting screen time before bed, you increase your chances of getting restful sleep.

Consider the benefits of constantly prioritizing your sleep: your body's natural mechanisms sync, promoting hunger regulation and contributing to a more stable blood sugar profile. By incorporating quality sleep as a key component of your diabetes management approach, you empower yourself to face each day with more well-being and control.

Fourteenth

Unleash the Power of Stress Management

In the complex tapestry of diabetes treatment, stress appears as a powerful component capable of influencing blood glucose levels. Combat potential surges by researching effective stress management practices that are compatible with your lifestyle.

Begin a journey of serenity with mindfulness techniques such as relaxing breathing exercises, yoga sessions, or meditation. These relaxation techniques not only relieve stress but also promote overall well-being.

Consider a situation in which, armed with these stress-relieving tools, you may navigate life's obstacles with renewed serenity. The effect goes beyond mere relaxation; it orchestrates a symphony of balance within your body, resulting in stable blood sugar levels. As you incorporate stress management into your diabetes care regimen, imagine a landscape in which tranquility complements glucose control, paving the road for a healthier, more empowered you.

Fifteenth Step to Take

Less salt, happy kidneys, cool pressure

Navigate the journey to better health with reduced salt intake for kidney health and blood pressure.

In the complicated dance of health management, salt intake is critical, regulating both kidney function and blood pressure levels. Take control of your health by embracing a purposeful reduction in dietary salt.

Choose fresh, unprocessed products that not only taste better but also help to protect the kidneys and regulate blood pressure. Transform your culinary adventures by flavoring with a symphony of herbs and spices, allowing you to explore new flavors without jeopardizing your health.

Consider a culinary landscape in which every savory bite not only satisfies your taste senses but also benefits your kidneys and lowers your blood pressure.

As you embark on this salt sensibility adventure, envision yourself becoming healthier and more balanced—a witness to the transformative power of mindful food choices.

Sixteenth

Navigate the healing path

Diabetes increases the risk of infection and hinders the healing process.

In the world of diabetes, alertness becomes your friend. Diabetes increases the risk of infection and slows the natural healing process, therefore treating bumps and bruises as soon as possible is critical.

If a minor mishap occurs, treat cuts and wounds right away. Maintain meticulous hygiene, and use antibiotic cream to create an atmosphere conducive to healing. Your vigilant eye serves as a buffer against unforeseen difficulties.

Extend this care to frequent foot exams, which are a ritual for detecting any tiny indicators of injury. In the delicate dance of diabetes and well-being, your dedication to quick treatment elevates each healing journey to a testament of perseverance.

Seventeenth

If you smoke, stopping is critical

In the complex tapestry of diabetes management, cutting ties with smoking appears as a critical thread. Smoking, a tenacious foe, exacerbates diabetic issues, particularly in terms of cardiovascular health.

Take control of your health by going on the journey to quit smoking. It's more than just a step; it's a leap toward protecting your cardiovascular and general health. Seek out the assistance and resources that speak to you, and carve a route that leads to greater freedom from the grip of smoking. Your lungs breathe easily, and your heart beats with a resilient rhythm.

Eighteenth

Power up with nutrient-dense foods

Include nutrient-dense foods such as berries, sweet potatoes, omega-3 fatty acid-rich fish, and dark leafy greens in your daily diet.

Increase your diabetes-fighting armory by incorporating a variety of superfoods.

Let berries, with their antioxidant properties, dance on your plate beside sweet potatoes,

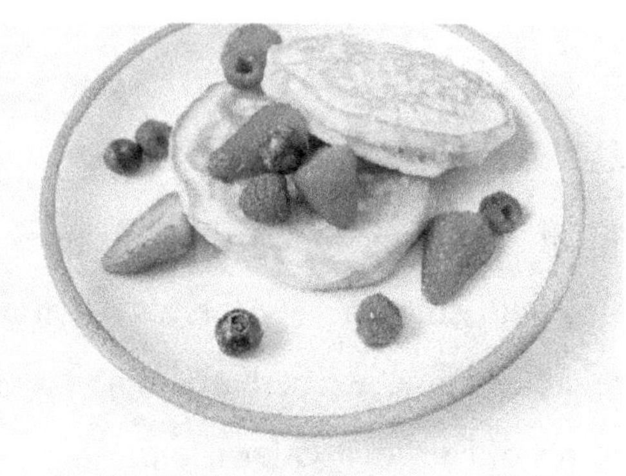

which are a rich source of minerals.

Navigate the ocean of omega-3 fatty acids with fish as an ally to improve heart health.

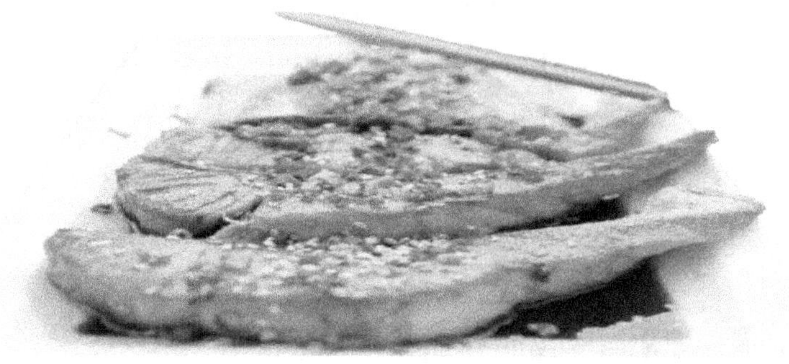

Allow dark leafy greens to reveal their nutritious magnificence, enhancing your meals. Prioritize quality while avoiding saturated and trans fats. Fuel your body with the vitality of superfoods to strengthen your defenses against diabetes's challenges.

Nineteenth

Navigate the medication maze

Gain a thorough understanding of blood glucose-lowering drugs.

Engage with your healthcare practitioner to understand the nuances of their effects, ideal dosage, potential side effects, and seamless integration into your overall management strategy. Illuminate the route to making well-informed decisions, ensuring that your medicine regimen is consistent with your diabetic journey.

Twentieth Step to Take

Navigating a diabetes friendly Diet

Follow an eating plan that helps you manage your diabetes.

Begin a dietary program designed to promote diabetic management. Reduce saturated fats, avoid trans fats, choose healthy oils, and maintain a balanced calorie intake. Consult your healthcare provider or a seasoned dietitian to create a personalized nutritional plan that corresponds with your diabetes control objectives. For example, replace deep-fried foods with grilled ones, use olive oil as a heart-healthy substitute, and eat nutrient-dense, low-calorie snacks to find the appropriate balance for your specific needs.

Twenty-First

Create your personal diabetes care schedule

Work with your primary care provider to create a specific care schedule.

Form a collaborative partnership with your primary care provider to create a bespoke care schedule that is precisely matched to your specific health needs. Immerse yourself in the routine of frequent blood sugar monitoring, persistently perform preventive testing, and create a proactive approach to strengthening your health fortress. By following this painstakingly planned program, you equip yourself to tackle the complexities of diabetic treatment with resilience and forethought.

Creating a personalized diabetes care regimen entails combining numerous variables to meet your specific health needs. Here's an in-depth look:

Regular Blood Sugar Monitoring: Schedule daily blood sugar readings, observing patterns after meals and at different times of day. If there is a surge, consider your recent meal choices and modify accordingly.

Preventive Tests: Collaborate with your healthcare team to plan routine A1c, lipid, and kidney function tests. These tests provide a comprehensive picture of your general health and help guide any changes to your treatment approach.

Nutritional Planning: Work with a dietician to develop a personalized food plan based on your interests and lifestyle. This could include modifying portion sizes, selecting the proper carbohydrate, protein, and fat ratio, and including foods that have a good impact on blood sugar.

Physical Activity Routine: Create a tailored training routine based on your fitness level and preferences. This could involve a combination of aerobic activities such as walking or swimming, strength training, and flexibility exercises. Regular physical activity improves insulin sensitivity and promotes general well-being.

Medication management: If medicine is part of your treatment plan, create a consistent regimen for taking prescribed medications. Communicate freely with your healthcare practitioner about any side effects or concerns, ensuring that modifications can be made as needed.

Stress Management Techniques: Incorporate stress-relieving activities into your daily routine, such as mindfulness meditation, deep breathing exercises, or indulging in hobbies that you enjoy. Regular stress management contributes to steady blood glucose levels.

Regular Check-Ins with the Healthcare Team: Set up regular evaluations with your healthcare team to examine progress, resolve issues, and make any required changes to your care plan. Open communication ensures that your care adapts to your changing health needs.

By incorporating these examples into your personalized diabetes care plan, you take a proactive approach to effectively managing diabetes and improving your overall well-being.

Twenty-Second

Link hearts: connect with others

Seek help from friends, family, and support groups.

Connecting with others is an important part of navigating the challenges of diabetes. Here's a thorough analysis with examples:

Family involvement: Example: Help your family understand your food preferences and encourage them to join you in living a healthy lifestyle. This not only creates a supportive workplace, but also makes diabetes management a team effort.

Friends serve as accountability partners: For example, share your fitness goals with your pals and invite them to participate in regular physical activity. Having a workout buddy not only makes exercise more fun, but it also fosters a sense of reciprocal accountability.

Support groups: Join a local or online diabetic support group to hear from others who have faced similar issues.

Participating in group discussions, whether in person or online, can provide emotional support, practical advice, and a sense of belonging.

Socializing mindfully: For example, when socializing, be open about your nutritional preferences with friends and colleagues. Choose eateries that have healthier options, and inform individuals around you about your condition to build a supportive social circle.

Virtual Connections: For example, use social media sites or diabetes-specific applications to engage with a larger community. This allows you to share ideas, learn about new management practices, and encourage others on the same road.

Educational Events: Attend diabetes management classes or seminars with friends or family. Learning together provides a common understanding of the illness and a collaborative approach to overall well-being.

Cooking Classes and Workshops: Consider taking cooking workshops focused on diabetic-friendly cuisine. Attend these workshops with friends or family to create a bonding experience focusing on eating a nutritious diet.

Family Challenges: For example, start a family exercise challenge or make a commitment to exploring new, healthy dishes together. This not only fosters a supportive environment, but it also makes diabetes management a positive and inclusive family activity.

Connecting with people not only provides emotional support, but it also allows for shared experiences, making the diabetes management journey more bearable and, at times, pleasurable.

Twenty-Third

Shop for diabetes supplies

Provide yourself with important diabetes supplies such as a blood glucose meter, test strips, a lancing device, lancets,

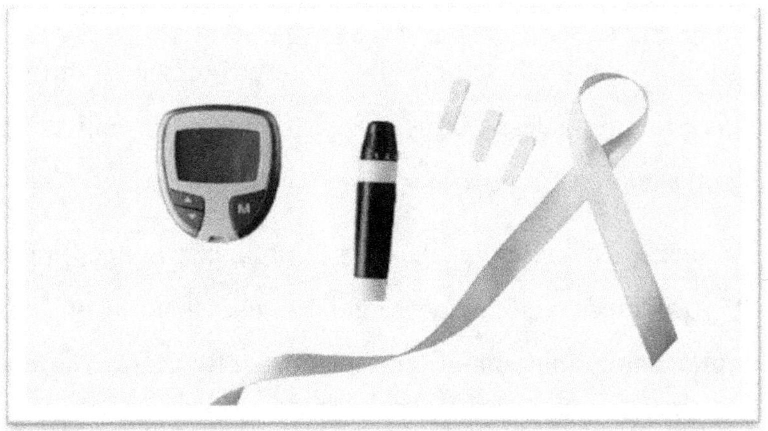

prescriptions, syringes, and sharps container.

Keep a journal or use a mobile app to track your progress.

Shopping for diabetes supplies is an important part of managing your illness effectively. Here is an example-based exploration:

Blood glucose meters: Choose a dependable blood glucose meter that is compatible with your lifestyle. Choose a model that includes memory storage and interoperability with mobile apps for easy tracking.

Test strips and lancets: Example: Make sure you have an adequate supply of test strips and lancets. Consider purchasing in bulk to save money and limit the number of shopping excursions.

Lancing device: Example - Choose a lancing device with customizable depth settings for more customized comfort. This provides a less obtrusive experience when collecting blood samples for glucose testing.

Medications: Example - Use a pill organizer to keep track of your meds and never forget to take them. Consider implementing automatic prescription refills to ensure a continuous supply.

Syringe and Sharps Container: Example - If insulin injections are part of your treatment plan, stock up on syringes and properly dispose of spent ones in a designated sharps container. Many pharmacies provide sharps disposal services for increased convenience.

Monitoring journal or app: Example - Use a diabetes management journal or a mobile app to record your blood sugar levels, meals, medications, and physical exercise. This thorough method offers vital insights to you and your healthcare team.

Emergency supplies: Example - Create a small diabetes emergency kit that includes fast-acting glucose, identification indicating your diabetes status, and emergency contact information. This ensures readiness for unexpected scenarios.

Regular inventory checks: Example - Create a process for checking your diabetes supply inventory. Set reminders to reorder things in advance to avoid disruptions in your daily management routine.

Travel-Friendly Supplies: Example - When traveling, bring a portable supply kit that includes all necessary things. Ensure that your blood glucose meter, prescriptions, and other supplies are easily accessible throughout your vacation.

Technology integration: Example: - Look into technological solutions that work with your supplies, such as Bluetooth-enabled glucose meters that sync data to your smartphone. This simplified technique improves the efficiency with which you track and manage diabetes.

Maintaining a well-stocked and structured supply inventory empowers you to continuously follow your diabetes care plan. Regular checks and technology integrations help to a more efficient and successful management experience.

Twenty-Fourth

Primary care provider to select

Choose a primary care physician that values individuality, listens to your concerns, and works with you to develop a complete treatment plan.

Selecting a primary care provider is an important step in your healthcare journey.

Here is an example-based exploration:

Respect for individuality: Example - Look for a primary care physician who understands your specific health needs and respects your personal preferences. A provider who considers your lifestyle, values, and goals helps to create a more tailored and effective treatment plan.

Active Listening: Example - Find a healthcare provider who actively listens to your issues and promotes open communication. This collaborative approach builds a trustworthy relationship, allowing you to share health facts and make educated decisions together.

A Comprehensive Treatment Plan: Example - Consult a primary care practitioner who prioritizes a thorough treatment plan. This should include regular check-ups, preventive tests, and a proactive approach to managing chronic illnesses such as diabetes. Regularly evaluating and revising the plan ensures that it remains relevant to your changing health needs.

Make Informed Decisions: Example - Select a healthcare practitioner who consults with you before making decisions.

This may include discussing alternative treatment options, describing potential advantages and dangers, and ensuring you have the necessary knowledge to make educated health decisions.

Accessible Lab Results: Example - Choose a provider who values quick communication of lab results. Accessible and open reporting keeps you informed about your health state, allowing you and your healthcare team to make any required changes to your treatment plan.

Progress monitoring: Example - Schedule regular progress meetings with your primary care provider. Assessing lab findings, discussing lifestyle modifications, and evaluating progress or problems ensure that your treatment plan continues effective. Adjustments can be made as necessary to improve your general health.

The Holistic Health Approach: Example - Consider a primary care clinician who believes in a holistic health approach. This entails addressing not only physical health but also psychological and emotional well-being. This approach recognizes the interconnection of several areas of your health.

Coordination of Care: Example - Look for a primary care physician who works closely with specialists and other healthcare providers involved in your treatment. This enables a consistent and comprehensive strategy, particularly if you have various health conditions.

Choosing the correct primary care practitioner is an important step toward proactive, patient-centered treatment. Prioritize attributes that are consistent with your tastes and values, resulting in a happy and collaborative healthcare partnership.

Twenty-Fifth Step to Take

Continuous self-education

Knowledge is your most potent instrument.

Continuously learning about diabetes is critical for good management. Here is an example-based exploration:

Read Diabetes Literature: Example - Review your healthcare team's educational materials on a regular basis. This could include brochures, booklets, and internet resources. Understanding the basics of diabetes, its complications, and management strategies allows you to make more informed health decisions.

Attend Educational Programs: Example - Actively attend diabetes-related workshops, seminars, or webinars. Participate in local or online educational sessions hosted by healthcare facilities, patient advocacy groups, or community centers. These events offer useful insights, practical recommendations, and the opportunity to meet with specialists and other diabetics.

Stay Informed of Developments: Example - Stay up to date on the newest advancements in diabetes research, technology, and treatment choices by following credible information sites on a regular basis. Subscribe to newsletters, read articles from medical magazines, and visit reputable health sites. Being aware of breakthroughs allows you to debate upcoming choices with your healthcare team.

Use Digital Apps and Tools: Example - Look at diabetes management apps and solutions that include educational content, tracking capabilities, and individualized insights. Many apps include daily suggestions, nutritional advice, and reminders for medication or blood sugar monitoring. Incorporating technology into your learning process can make material more accessible and useful.

Ask questions during healthcare visits: Example - Actively engage in talks with your healthcare staff during appointments. Please do not hesitate to ask questions about your disease, treatment options, or lifestyle changes. Understanding the reasons behind recommendations improves your ability to manage diabetes successfully.

Seek Guidance from Certified Diabetes Educators: Example - Contact qualified diabetes educators for specialized advice. These individuals specialize in diabetes education and may provide personalized knowledge depending on your specific requirements. Work with them to develop a complete self-management plan.

Read personal stories and experiences: Example - Look into books, blogs, or articles published by people who relate their personal experiences with diabetes. Learning from real-life experiences can provide practical insights and motivational stories that are relevant to your own struggles and accomplishments.

Continuous education provides you with the knowledge and skills necessary to negotiate the difficulties of diabetes. By being informed and involved, you become an active participant in your healthcare journey, which helps to improve diabetes management and general well-being.

Remember that managing diabetes is a continual process. Stay proactive, informed, and connected in order to live a

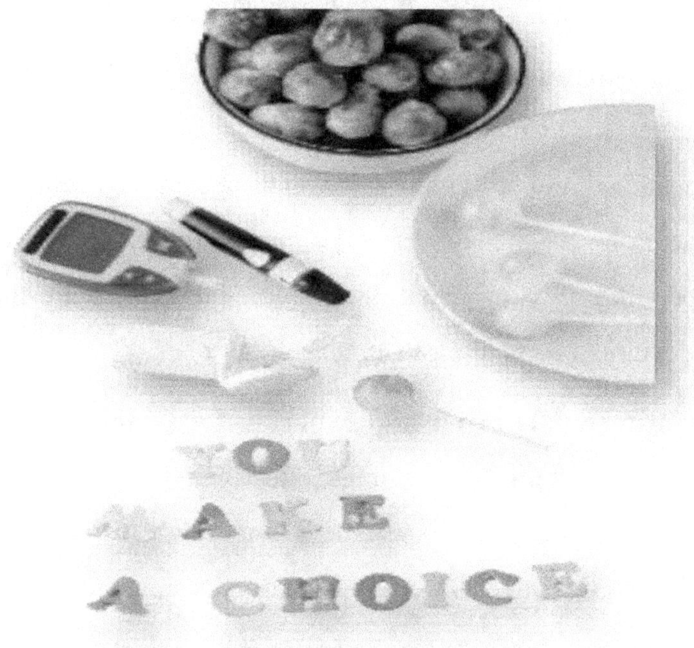

healthy and joyful life with diabetes.

CHAPTER 3

Tackle Troubles: Prevent Complications

Alright, friends, let's have a heart-to-heart regarding diabetic complications. Now, I'm not going to throw a lot of fancy terms at you. I'm keeping things genuine, like speaking with a buddy at the neighborhood restaurant.

So, here's the deal: diabetes may stir up some health difficulties, no question. But guess what? You've got the capacity to sidestep these issues or at least press the snooze button on them. I'm talking about tag-alongs like heart disease, renal troubles, funky nerves, and other worries like foot problems, oral challenges, fuzzy vision, hearing glitches, and a little of mental health drama.

Now, don't you worry – I'm not just here to spill the tea; I'm here with answers. Learn the ropes on avoiding or postponing these diabetic sidekicks and sprinkle a little magic on your general health.

This isn't rocket science; it's more like your grandma's tried-and-true treatments. Let's get in and keep it easy, just like trading recipes over Sunday brunch. 🌞 📱

Diabetes and Your Heart: Taking Care of the Beat

So, let's speak about diabetes and your heart. They're sort of like companions that typically tag around together. But the good news? You have the ability to defend your heart and control diabetes with some easy lifestyle modifications. It's a little like a two-for-one bargain.

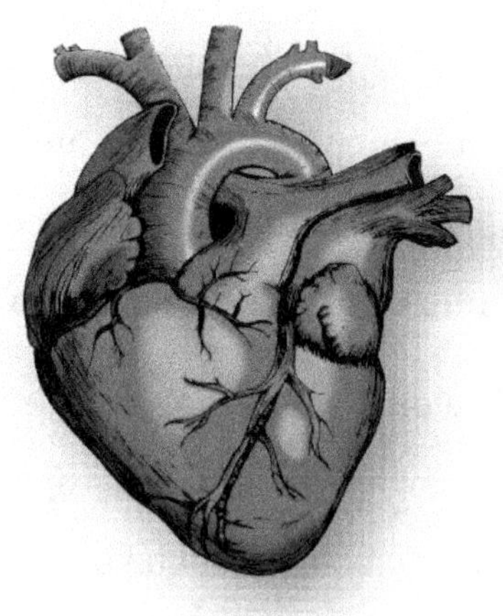

Regular checkups are your heart's BFF

Now, here's the actual talk: heart disease is a major concern. It's the biggest cause of both women and men kicking the bucket in the U.S. And if you've got diabetes, you're in the line of fire - twice as likely to get heart disease or a stroke, and at an earlier age. But wait on, it's not all doom and gloom. Changing a few items in your regular routine may lessen the risk of heart disease and give your heart a boost. Plus, it helps you control diabetes like an expert.

Let's break it down. Heart disease isn't just one issue; it's like a family of disorders playing with your heart. You've got your superstar, coronary artery disease, creating issues by blocking up blood flow. Picture it as sludge in your pipes — not enjoyable. But that's not all; it may develop in other body regions, too, as in your legs, calling itself peripheral arterial disease (PAD). Sneaky, right?

Now, here's where diabetes comes into play. Over time, elevated blood sugar may be a major nuisance, damage your heart's pals — the blood arteries and nerves. It also brings along certain companions that boost the risk of heart disease, such high blood pressure and cholesterol troubles.

Sneaky, but we've got techniques to identify them using blood pressure checks and basic blood tests.

But wait, there's more. Smoking, being a touch too round, missing the exercise party, and snacking on the incorrect foods may also join the heart-hurting team. And let's not forget about too much drink — it's like inviting trouble around.

Diabetes also raises your risk of heart failure. It's not about your heart giving up; it's more about striving to execute its job correctly.

This might lead to swelling legs and difficulties breathing. Not cool, right? But catch it early, and you've got a chance at halting or slowing down the problem.

Now, let's discuss exams. Checking your blood pressure, cholesterol levels, and weight is like giving your heart a check-up. Your doctor could prescribe more tests, such an ECG or EKG to monitor your heart's electrical feel or an echocardiography to see how thick your heart muscles are. There's also the Treadmill Test — not for cardio, but to assess how your heart handles an exercise.

So, what's the game plan? Easy.

- Eat Smart: Load up on fresh fruits, vegetables, lean protein, and nutritious grains. Ditch the processed munchies and go easy on the sugary beverages and liquor.

- Keep It Light: Shedding even a little of weight may do wonders. Think 5-7% of your body weight — like lowering 10 to 14 pounds if you're around 200.

- Move Your Body: Get your groove on with at least 150 minutes a week of moderate-intensity exercise. It's like a love song for your heart.

- ABCs Check: Keep checks on your A1C levels, blood pressure below 140/90 mm Hg, and control cholesterol levels. Oh, and remove the smoking habit — it's a deal-breaker.

- Chill Out: Stress is a mood-killer for your heart. Try relaxing with a counselor, meditation, a quick stroll, or some good old family and friend vibes.

And hey, if your doctor prescribes certain medicines, it's like giving your heart a little additional support.

Last item - partner up with a diabetic educator. They're like your own guides to averting health difficulties, particularly heart-related ones. So, go ahead, take care of your heart. Your actual MVP on this adventure. If you haven't met a diabetes educator yet, push your GP for the connection.

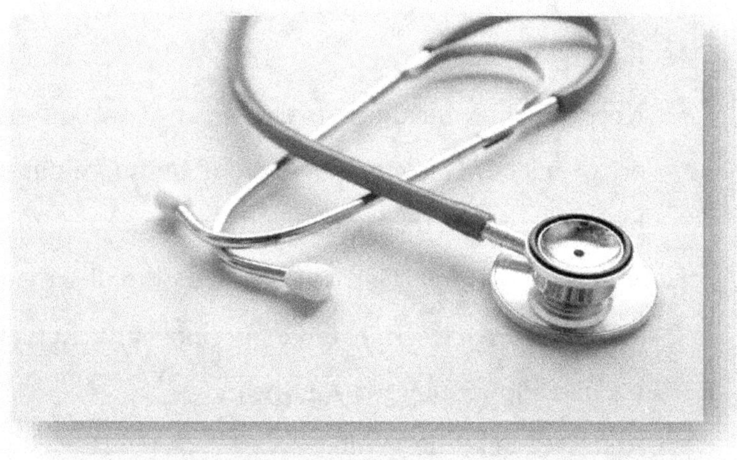

Regular checkups are your heart's BFF - don't miss 'em! Here's to a healthy heart and an easier journey with diabetes. You've got this! 🖤 ✨

Diabetes and Chronic Kidney Disease

Let's discuss a very important topic: kidneys. These days, they operate silently until a hiccup occurs, like backstage heroes. You should watch these superstars closely, especially if you have diabetes.

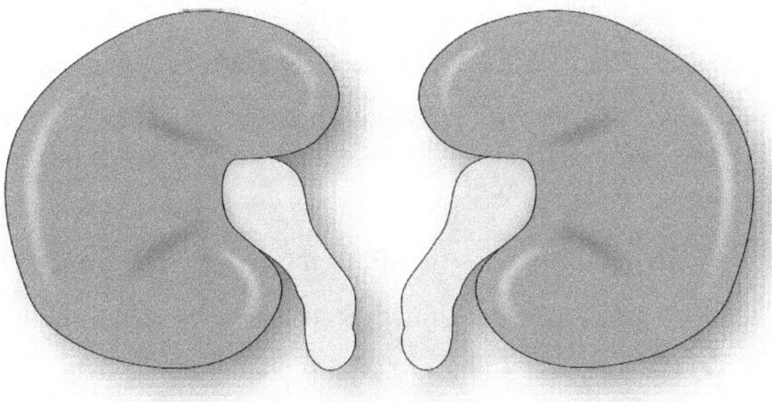

The sneaky ninja that is Chronic Kidney Disease (CKD) is what it is called. It approaches cautiously and frequently gives no notice. Until it throws a full-blown fiesta and you require dialysis or a kidney transplant to keep the show going, you might not even notice it's crashed the party.

The bottom line for those on the diabetes team is to make sure your kidneys receive routine examinations. Simple tests such as blood and urine can be used by your doctor to perform magic. Catching chronic kidney disease (CKD) early enough to prevent it from becoming worse is similar to getting an annual check-up for your kidneys.

Here's a fun fact: diabetes and CKD get along well. This tag-along buddy is present in about 1 in 3 persons with diabetes. Diabetic kidney disease (DKA) can cause kidney problems regardless of the kind of diabetes you have.

It's important to state that:

- kidney disease is the ninth most common cause of mortality in the United States, which makes them sly.
- approximately, one in three diabetic warriors is said to have CKD.
- every day, 170 diabetics start kidney failure treatment.

The following summarizes the way that diabetes and renal disease work together: Your kidneys' nephrons, which are small filters, get upset when high blood sugar decides to throw a little party. It irritates blood vessels and overstays its welcome over time. It is comparable to that rowdy visitor who refuses to go.

The early stages of CKD are frequently characterized by a slow rate of development. Pretty cunning, huh? Consequently, unless your physician opens the door for a check-up, you won't even be aware that it's there.

You can protect your kidneys by acting as their protector, though—this is your superpower! Like an expert, control your blood pressure, cholesterol, and sugar levels. It is not only a strong plan for your heart and blood arteries, but it is also excellent for your kidneys. Following all, elevated blood pressure, cholesterol, and blood sugar levels are similar to the triple threat that results in heart attacks and strokes.

Here are some kidney-friendly suggestions to get you started:

- Maintaining proper blood sugar levels will benefit your kidneys.
- At least twice a year, schedule an A1C test. Discuss what is most effective for you with your doctor.

- Monitor your blood pressure and try to keep it around 140/90 mmHg. This one can be helped by both medication and lifestyle modifications.
- Remain in the comfort zone for your cholesterol.
- Reduce your intake of sodium because salt is bad for your kidneys.
- Fill your dish with assorted fruits and vegetables.
- Transfer that body! When it comes to kidney health, regular exercise is like a dance party.
- Adhere to the prescribed dosage — it's an essential component of your superhero regimen.

Warning to individuals who belong to the prediabetes club

You're protecting your kidneys by preventing type 2 diabetes. An individual weighing 200 pounds, for example, might lose 10 to 14 pounds, or 5% to 7% of their total weight, according to studies. 150 minutes a week of moderate exercise combined with a healthy diet? This is yours!

To summarize: exercising, eating healthily, and maintaining an active lifestyle can help you keep your kidneys functioning properly!

Mind Matters: Diabetes and Mental Health

Now let's discus diabetes and mental health. It's not just about blood sugar levels; it's also about your thoughts, emotions, and approach to life's obstacles. Think of it as your diabetes journey's backstage crew. The truth is that mental health issues can throw you off, which makes following your diabetes treatment plan a little more difficult.

Let's talk about the mind-body link. Your body's level of health is influenced by your ideas, emotions, and beliefs. Diabetes may become slightly more problematic if you are also coping with untreated mental health concerns, and vice versa. The favorable tidings? When one gets better, the other usually does too.

Let's raise awareness about depression, which goes beyond being in a foul mood. It's a medical disorder that might make you feel hopeless and less interested in activities you used to enjoy. The plot twist is that it can also interfere with your diabetes management, increasing your risk of consequences like nerve damage and heart disease.

Are you aware? Depression is two to three times as common in those with diabetes. The problematic issue is that only 25–50% of them receive a diagnosis and course of treatment. The clever move, though, comes here: therapy, medication, or a combination of the two, is typically a rather effective kind of treatment. Disregarding it? Usually, though, that makes matters worse rather than better. A wide range of symptoms are associated with depression, including:

- Feeling depressed or meaningless
- Losing enthusiasm for hobbies or pastimes
- Overeating or not wanting to eat at all
- Sleeping too much or not being able to sleep at all
- Having difficulty focusing or making choices
- I'm exhausted.
- Feeling angry, nervous, despondent, or guilty
- Experiencing headaches, cramps, aches, or stomach issues
- Having suicidal or fatal thoughts

If you suspect depression is knocking on your door, reach out to your doctor pronto. Early treatment is the superhero cape you need for a better quality of life.

Now, stress and anxiety – they're like unwelcome guests crashing your party. They mess with your daily care routine and can send your blood sugar levels on a rollercoaster ride. Managing diabetes while juggling long-term conditions can be a source of anxiety. The good news? Therapy usually steals the spotlight over medicine, and a mix of both might be the winning combo.

Are you under stress? Relaxation techniques, a brisk walk, or a conversation with a friend can all be very beneficial. For a smoother journey, cut back on caffeine and alcohol, eat well, and get those Zs. Has diabetes ever made you feel overwhelmed? That is the misery of diabetes. It's as though diabetes is taking over and you're fed up with the show. In an 18-month period, it affects between 33% to 50% of diabetics, making it a rather prevalent occurrence.

The catch is that it is not treated by medication for conditions like anxiety or depression. As an alternative, collaborate with a diabetes educator, mental health therapist, or endocrinologist. Join a support group, make tiny goals, and together, let's reclaim control. Don't forget your health care team – they are always there to assist you. Speak up if the rollercoaster of mental health is getting to you. Help is available and you're not alone—just have a chat!

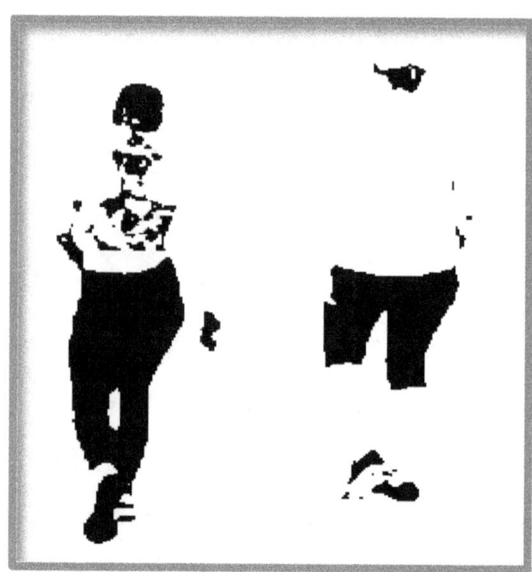

Brisk walk is helpful in stress management

Diabetes and Nerve Damage

Let us discuss the significance of controlling your blood sugar levels – not only for day-to-day tasks but also to avert major surprises in the future.

Has nerve damage ever occurred to you? It's one probable side effect of persistently elevated blood sugar levels. Imagine a situation in which elevated blood sugar acts as a scoundrel, causing harm to your nerves and interfering with messages to different areas of your body. The outcome? Anything that can interfere with your regular routine, from little numbness to pain.

And what about it? Approximately 50% of people with diabetes experience nerve damage. The good news is that you can avoid it altogether or at least postpone it if you maintain a healthy blood sugar level. Extra? You'll experience improved energy and general well-being!

Nerve damage is a slow-moving disease that doesn't strike like a storm. Thus, the key is to identify those symptoms early on. Let's now discuss the sneak-peek symptoms and the four primary categories of nerve injury.

Peripheral Nerve Damage is first. You may be with this if you have ever felt like there are "pins and needles", or tingling in your feet. Or if your feet appear extremely sensitive. It can cause pain, numbness, and even more serious foot issues. Usually, it begins in the feet.

Damage to the Autonomic Nerves, which can affect your heart, bladder, stomach, intestines, sex organs, or eyes, comes next on the list. This one can cause a lot of difficulties, ranging from bladder issues to adjustments in how your eyes respond to light.

Legs, buttocks, hips, and thighs suffer from **Proximal Nerve Injury**. You may be familiar with severe discomfort and difficulty getting out of a sitting position.

Finally, damage to individual nerves known as **Focal Nerve Injury**. Consider experiencing headaches behind one eye, hand weakness, or difficulty focusing.

Let's now discuss risk factors. Nerve damage can happen to anybody with diabetes, but certain circumstances make it more likely. A number of factors can tip the scales, including difficult blood sugar levels, the length of diabetes, age over 40, being overweight, and high blood pressure or cholesterol.

Advice for prevention? Maintain proper blood pressure control, exercise, lose weight if necessary, cut back on alcohol, quit smoking, maintain a nutritious diet, and take your medications as directed.

What time is best to call your doctor? If you detect changes in your digestion, urine, or sexual function, if you feel lightheaded or faint, or if you see a wound or sore on your foot that is not acting well. Being aware of these symptoms early on can have a profound impact.

Remeber that you have the power. Nerve injury can be prevented with vigilantism, frequent foot care, and check-ups with the doctor. You are responsible for your own health! 🌟💪

Diabetes and Your Feet, Oral Health, Hearing, and Vision Well-Being

Alright, managing diabetes is like juggling a lot of balls— blood sugar checks, healthy eating, staying active, meds, doctor's visits… but here's the thing, don't let your **Feet** be the forgotten ball in the juggle. Daily care is your best defense against foot complications.

Now, about half of folks with diabetes deal with nerve damage, often in the feet and legs. Some feel numbness or pain, others, nothing at all. Yeah, no pain sounds great, but it's a double-edged sword. Without it, you might miss issues like cuts or sores. Catching problems early by checking your feet daily is a game-changer and significantly lowers the risk of amputation.

Risk factors for nerve damage? Tricky blood sugar, longtime diabetes, age over 40, being overweight, high blood pressure, and cholesterol. Keep blood sugar in check, and follow good habits like not smoking, eating healthy, staying active, and taking meds.

Now, let's talk foot care. Daily checks, gentle washing, comfy shoes, trimmed toenails, and regular foot doc visits are your allies. Keep that blood flowing, choose feet-friendly activities, and when in doubt, ask your doc about keeping those feet happy.

Next up, **Oral Health.** Taking care of your teeth is a big deal. For those with diabetes, it's even more critical because high blood sugar weakens infection-fighting white blood cells. Manage diabetes, manage gum disease. So, brush and floss regularly, see your dentist, and shout it out if you have diabetes—it's vital info for them.

Now, **The Ears**. Did you know diabetes could play tricks on your hearing? High and low blood sugar levels can damage those inner ear nerves. Hearing loss is twice as common in folks with diabetes. Watch for signs—asking others to repeat, trouble in noisy places, or cranking up the volume. Protect your ears: control blood sugar, check your hearing yearly, avoid loud noises, and chat with your doctor about hearing-friendly meds.

Last but not least, **Vision**. Diabetes can cause diabetic retinopathy, a leading cause of blindness. Longer diabetes duration, high blood sugar, and smoking up the risk. Regular eye checks, controlling blood sugar, pressure, and cholesterol, quitting smoking, and staying active are your vision heroes.

Remember, you're the superhero in your diabetes journey. Keep those feet tapping, smile shining, ears tuned in, and eyes sparkling! ✳️ 🤍

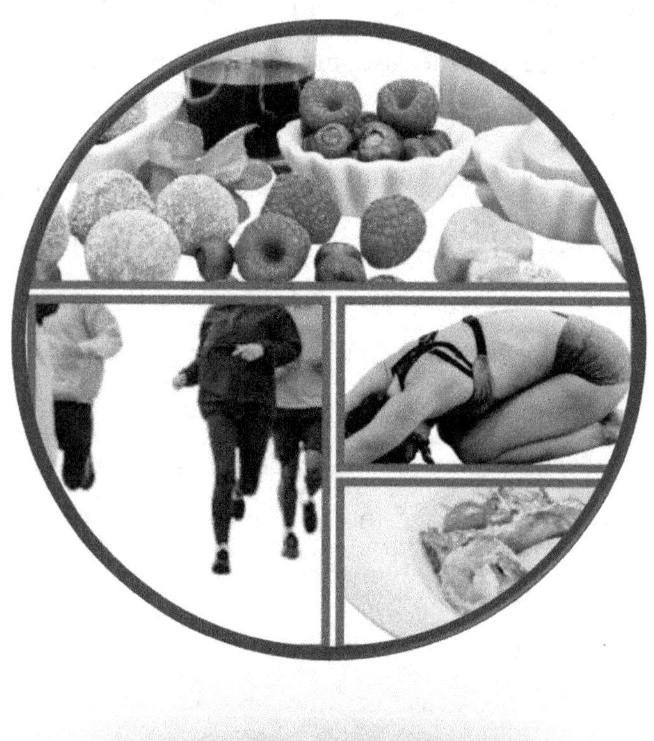

Smart eating, regular exercise, and embracing a healthy lifestyle are pivotal for managing diabetes and warding off complications.

CHAPTER 4

Comprehensive List of Diabetic Foods to Eat and Avoid

Consider this a grocery shopping guide to help you select which foods are healthy to consume and which to avoid if you have diabetes.

Planning and replanning your food list is especially beneficial while eating for type 2 diabetes.

Creating a meal and snack plan with delicious, balanced foods will help you remain on track and improve your overall health. You may prevent food waste and save money by going grocery shopping with a list you've created while keeping your budget and meal planning in mind.

So, which foods should you buy from the shop and which should you avoid?

Consume only certain foods.

Packaged foods can still be included in your diet; just make informed choices. Read the Nutrition Facts label and ingredient list to become an informed consumer who makes health-promoting food choices.

Simply because a product is labeled as "natural" does not imply that it is fundamentally superior. The back of the packages will provide you with the information you need to make a decision. Look for the serving size, which specifies how much food is in one dish.

Take note of the amount of saturated fat, salt, and added sugar. Ideally, these percentages should fall between 7% and 10% of the Daily Value. The Daily Value indicates how much of each nutrient is available in a single serving of food; 5% or less is considered low, whereas 20% or more is considered excessive. Keep track of the dish's total carbohydrates and look for sugar in the ingredients.

A diabetic diet might consist of any dietary item. However, you should limit your intake of certain foods.

Limit your consumption of the foods listed below:

- Sugar-sweetened beverages, such as soda and sports drinks.
- Baked products and pastries in packages.

- Refined grains, such as white bread (rather, use whole grains).
- Sweetened fruits (search for unsweetened dry, canned, or frozen fruits).
- Hotdogs, sausages, and bacon are all processed meats.

Healthy staples to include:

So, what should you be producing more of? Prioritize whole, minimally processed meals. Whole grains are richer in fiber and minerals than processed grains. Your diet should be mostly made up of vegetables, fruits, whole grains, legumes, healthy proteins, and healthy fats.

Making comprehensive grocery and pantry lists centered on staple meals and any specialty items will make shopping much easier. Meal planning and batch cooking can help you save time and energy in the kitchen. To consume healthful meals, you must first stock your pantry with them.

Vegetables

Most of us do not consume enough vegetables. They are rich in vitamins, minerals, and antioxidants. Vegetables are often classified into two types: starchy and non-starchy.

Starchy veggies have more carbohydrates (around 15 grams per 1/2 cup cooked), so keep that in mind when planning your menu. Consume a wide range of veggies to acquire a variety of nutrients. Fresh vegetables taste wonderful. Frozen and canned meals are also wonderful options because they are less expensive and last longer; however, keep an eye on the sodium levels.

Non-starchy vegetables list

Certainly, let's review the list of non-starchy vegetables:

1. Spinach
2. Kale
3. Collard
4. Swiss chard
5. Mustard greens
6. Carrots
7. Bell peppers
8. Cauliflower
9. Broccoli
10. Brussels sprouts
11. Asparagus
12. Celery
13. Tomatoes
14. Zucchini
15. Garlic
16. Onions
17. Mushroom
18. Okra
19. Cucumber
20. Eggplant
21. Artichoke
22. Green beans
23. Radishes
24. Snap peas

Starchy vegetables list

1. Winter squash
2. Sweet potatoes
3. Cassava
4. Yuca
5. Corn
6. Pumpkin
7. Sweet peas
8. Butternut squash
9. Acorn squash
10. Plantains
11. Beets
12. Parsnips
13. Rutabaga
14. Turnips
15. Spaghetti squash

Fruit

Fruit is a great option for diabetes. They are high in minerals and carbs (around 15 grams per serving). Fruit contains fiber, which can help reduce blood sugar levels.

Do not be afraid to ingest frozen fruit. They are frequently collected at the height of the growing season, making them as nutritious as fresh food. They will also last longer because they are frozen. If you have extra freezer space, consider purchasing the bags in bulk when they are on sale. Frozen fruits are fantastic in smoothies, porridge, or yogurt.

Fruits list

1. Apples
2. Bananas
3. Lemons
4. Limes
5. Plums
6. Apricots
7. Peaches
8. Strawberries
9. Blueberries
10. Citrus fruits (grapes, oranges, clementines)
11. Mangoes
12. Pineapple
13. Watermelon
14. Kiwi
15. Cherries
16. Raspberries
17. Blackberries
18. Papaya
19. Grapefruit
20. Cranberries

The fruits listed above are all diabetes-friendly and can be included in a diabetes-friendly diet when consumed in moderation and as part of a well-balanced meal plan.

Know that moderation is key, and it's advisable for individuals with diabetes to monitor their carbohydrate intake, considering the overall balance of their diet.

Beans

When you buy dry beans in quantity, they become one of the most affordable healthful meals available.

They take more time and effort to prepare, but they are far less expensive than many other protein sources.

Using an instant pot (pressure cooker) can save you time in the kitchen. Even in canned form, they remain inexpensive. A 1/3-cup portion of cooked beans contains around 15 grams of carbohydrates, and offers fiber, plant-based protein, and a variety of nutrients.

Beans list

1. Black beans.
2. Butterbeans
3. Chickpeas
4. Fava beans
5. Lima beans
6. Pinto beans
7. Navy beans
8. Kidney beans
9. Cannellini beans
10. Garbanzo beans
11. Black-eyed peas
12. Red kidney beans
13. Great Northern beans

All the beans in the above list are generally considered diabetes-friendly. However, individual responses to foods can vary, so it's always advisable to monitor blood sugar levels and consult with a healthcare professional or dietitian for personalized guidance based on specific health needs.

Grains

When you have diabetes, you can still consume grains and other simple carbohydrates. You should consume at least 50% whole grains. Also, keep track of your portion sizes. A 1/3-cup serving of cooked grains contains around 15 grams of carbs. A variety of non-starchy vegetables can help to fill you up.

Grains list

1. Rice (black, brown, and red)
2. Quinoa
3. Barley
4. Bean-Based Pasta (e.g., lentil, chickpea, black bean)
5. Whole wheat, or alternative grain-based (e.g., quinoa, brown rice).
6. Bread (one slice) Look for 100% whole grain or wheat.

Protein

Leaner beef slices can help reduce saturated fat. Try to consume a range of proteins, including seafood, twice each week. The vast majority of the animal proteins listed here contain zero grams of carbs.

However, you should not consume too much protein. A cooked piece of meat normally weighs between 3 and 4 ounces.

Protein list

1. Eggs
2. Fish
3. Seafood (salmon, haddock, cod, scallops, sardines, tuna)
4. Poultry (chicken breast, chicken thighs, ground chicken, turkey)
5. Red meat (beef tenderloin, cubed beef, flank steak, lean ground beef, sirloin)
6. Pork (pork loin, pork chops, ground pork)

Dairy

Dairy contains carbs. A cup of milk or yogurt has roughly 12 grams. Dairy products do, however, include protein, calcium, and vitamin D. If you want to reduce your saturated fat intake, stick to low-fat or fat-free dairy. Otherwise, flavored dairy products, such as flavored yogurts and milk, should be avoided because the additional sugars can significantly increase carbohydrate intake. Instead, choose for plain, unsweetened yogurt and other dairy products, and if necessary, top with fruit. Cheeses have fewer carbs than ordinary milk, but more protein and fat.

Diary list

1. Milk
2. Cheese (Cheddar and Swiss)
3. Plain yogurt
4. Cottage cheese

Nuts and Seeds

Nuts and seeds add healthful fats and plant-based protein to your diet while containing few carbs.

When feasible, choose low- or no-sodium foods. Nuts and seeds are excellent snacks or toppings for porridge and salads.

Nuts and Seeds list

1. Almonds
2. Walnuts
3. Hazelnuts
4. Chia seed
5. Pecans
6. Pistachios
7. Peanuts
8. Flaxseed
9. Hemp seeds
10. Sunflower seeds
11. Pumpkin seeds (pepitas)
12. Sesame seeds
13. Macadamia nuts
14. Cashews

Remember to choose unsalted and, if possible, raw or dry-roasted options to minimize added sodium and unhealthy fats.

In summary, diabetics may find grocery shopping terrifying, but it does not have to be.

To make things easier, make your shopping trip on a non-peak day. Many stores now provide grocery delivery, saving you a lot of time. Learning which foods to add into your diet more frequently will help you eat more efficiently, and the ingredients listed above can be combined to create a variety of great meals.

Read labels and look for bargains, but don't forget to have fun and experiment with the food you bring home.

CHAPTER 5

Nurturing Your Blood Sugar Naturally

This is essential for those suffering from diabetes and those who want to prevent it.

Naturally balancing your blood sugar levels not only prevents diabetes but also support those who have been diagnosed with it.

In this section, we take a look at a number of lifestyle and nutritional habits that promote healthy blood sugar levels. By using a holistic approach, you allow yourself to make informed decisions that promote your overall well-being.

Every facet of creating a harmonious relationship with your body's glucose balance is vital, from regular exercise routines to eating nutrient-rich foods.

Join me on this educational journey as we find natural strategies to balance your blood sugar levels. Your health is your most valuable asset, and with these insights, you'll be able to take care of it appropriately.

Let us work together to prevent diabetes and promote the well-being of those affected by it.

Exercise: Regular exercise, such as brisk walking, weightlifting, or dancing, can help with insulin sensitivity and blood sugar utilization. Include "exercise snacks" - quick bursts of activity throughout the day, such as mild walking or resistance workouts.

Manage Carb Intake: Just like I stated in the previous sections, plan your meals and keep track of your carb intake. Instead of processed foods, choose healthful grains like brown rice and quinoa. Sweet potatoes, for example, are better for managing blood sugar than regular potatoes.

Eat More Fiber: Consume fiber-rich foods such as vegetables, fruits, legumes, and whole grains. Beans and lentils, for example, can provide fiber as well as important minerals for improved blood sugar control.

Low Glycemic Index Meals

To help manage blood sugar, eat meals with a low glycemic index. Whole wheat pasta, non-starchy vegetables such as broccoli and cauliflower, and unsweetened Greek yogurt are also healthy choices.

Yoga: Practice yoga, meditation, or deep breathing exercises to reduce stress. Mindfulness-based stress reduction techniques, for example, can aid in management of stress and regulate blood sugar.

Portable Glucose Meter: Always use a portable glucose meter to examine your blood sugar levels. Keep track of your readings before and after you eat or exercise. This teaches you how 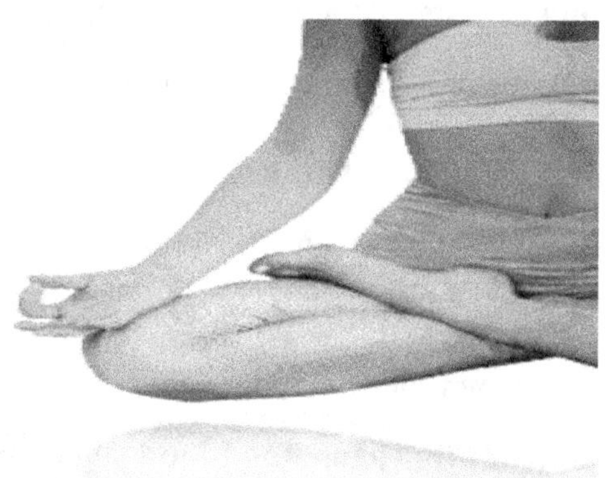 various activities and foods affect your blood sugar.

Get Enough Sleep: Aim for 7-8 hours of good sleep every night. Establish a bedtime routine and a comfortable sleeping environment by adjusting the room temperature and minimizing screen time before bedtime.

Foods High in Chromium and Magnesium: Incorporate nuts and whole grains high in chromium into your everyday diet. Dark leafy greens, such as spinach and almonds, are abundant in magnesium, which helps regulate blood sugar levels.

Incorporate Specific Foods into Your Diet: Try adding apple cider vinegar in salad dressings or cinnamon in oatmeal. However, before introducing these into your regimen, consult your doctor, especially if you are using blood sugar-lowering medications.

Maintain a Moderate Weight: Make long-term dietary changes to achieve moderate weight loss. For example, choose nutrient-dense foods like lean proteins, vegetables, and whole grains.

Increase Healthy Snack Frequency: Plan small, nutritious snacks in between meals. A handful of almonds, a piece of fruit, or Greek yogurt will help reduce excessive blood sugar fluctuations throughout the day.

Probiotic-rich Foods: Incorporate probiotic-rich foods like yogurt and sauerkraut into your daily diet. These can help with gut health, potentially contributing to better control of blood sugar over time.

Water:

Drink plenty of water and zero-calorie beverages to stay hydrated. This may reduce

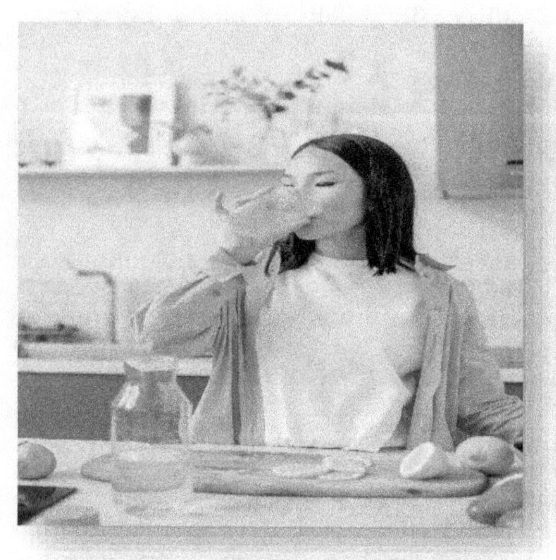

blood sugar levels and hence the risk of diabetes. Sugar-sweetened beverages should be avoided because they can raise blood glucose levels.

Incorporate these precise strategies into your daily practice to start your own road toward naturally balanced blood sugar.

CHAPTER 6

FAQs

Question: What is diabetes?

A: Diabetes is a chronic illness characterized by high blood sugar levels. It happens when the body either generates insufficient insulin (Type 1) or is unable to adequately use the insulin it produces (Type 2).

Q: What are some common signs of diabetes?

A: Common symptoms include excessive thirst, frequent urination, unexplained weight loss, lethargy, impaired eyesight, and poor wound healing.

Q: Is diabetes hereditary?

A: Yes, having a family history of diabetes increases the risk. Both genetic and environmental factors influence its growth.

Q: What is insulin, and why is it necessary for diabetes?

A: Insulin is a hormone that regulates blood sugar. Diabetes occurs when the body either produces insufficient insulin or is unable to use it adequately, resulting in high blood sugar levels.

Q: Can diabetes be prevented?

A: While not all types of diabetes can be avoided, lifestyle habits such as eating a nutritious diet, exercising regularly, and managing weight can help minimize the incidence of Type 2 diabetes.

Q: What is the distinction between Type I and Type II diabetes?

A: Type 1 diabetes is an autoimmune illness in which the body fails to manufacture insulin. Insulin resistance, or inadequate insulin production, is a defining feature of type 2 diabetes.

Q: How is diabetes diagnosed?

A: Blood tests used to diagnose diabetes include fasting blood sugar, oral glucose tolerance, and glycated hemoglobin (HbA1c) values.

Q: What is HbA1c, and why does it matter?

A: HbA1c is a blood test that measures average blood sugar levels over the last two to three months. It provides a long-term perspective on blood sugar regulation.

9. **Q**: Can diabetes be treated without medication?

A: Lifestyle changes, such as a healthy diet and frequent exercise, are essential for treating diabetes. In certain circumstances, medicine or insulin may be prescribed.

Q: How frequently should blood sugar be measured?

A: The frequency depends on the kind of diabetes and the individual's health requirements. Monitoring can occur several times each day or less frequently.

Q: Can diabetes cause complications?

A: Yes, diabetes can cause consequences such as heart disease, kidney damage, nerve difficulties, and vision loss.

Q: Are there diabetes-specific diets?

A: Diets should emphasize balanced nutrition, portion control, and carbohydrate tracking. Consultation with a dietitian is beneficial.

Q: How frequent is gestational diabetes, and how does it resolve after pregnancy?

A: Gestational diabetes develops throughout pregnancy. Women who have gestational diabetes are more likely to develop Type 2 diabetes, even though it usually cures after childbirth.

Q: Can alcohol be consumed by diabetics?

A: Moderate alcohol consumption is permitted, but it is critical to check blood sugar levels and be mindful of potential drug interactions.

Q: Is there a cure for diabetes?

A: There is no cure, but with careful management, diabetics can live healthy and fulfilling lives. New therapy possibilities are still being investigated through research.

CONCLUSION

To recap, living with diabetes is a journey fraught with decisions and concerns, but with information and a proactive approach, people can take control of their health and well-being. Embracing a complete strategy that encompasses food, exercise, emotional well-being, and informed healthcare decisions allows people to survive despite having diabetes.

The journey begins with identifying and understanding the emotional components of diabetes, dispelling myths, and accepting the reality of living with the disease. The next stage is to develop a comprehensive health plan that incorporates practical lifestyle changes.

Understanding the importance of dietary selection is critical. Adopting the Diabetes Plate Method, choosing carbohydrates wisely, and paying attention to portion sizes all contribute to good blood sugar regulation. Consuming nutrient-dense foods, such as vegetables, fruits, legumes, whole grains, lean proteins, diabetic-friendly dairy, and seeds/nuts, benefits overall health.

A focus on lifestyle factors such as weight management, enough sleep, stress management, and regular physical activity is crucial for balancing blood sugar and minimizing complications. Furthermore, careful blood sugar monitoring, adherence to medication regimens, and communication with healthcare professionals for individualized advice all contribute significantly to long-term well-being.

As people embark on their journeys to better living, joining a supportive group, staying educated through continuous education, and using modern tools to track progress become critical resources. Every aspect of diabetes management, from grocery shopping strategies to meal planning and the importance of frequent health exams, adds to a healthy and pleasurable lifestyle.

In summary, this book is a comprehensive guide that provides practical ideas, effective solutions, and a wealth of knowledge to assist people on their diabetic journey. Individuals can manage diabetes well while still living busy and joyful lives by making informed decisions, adopting a proactive mindset, and utilizing available resources.

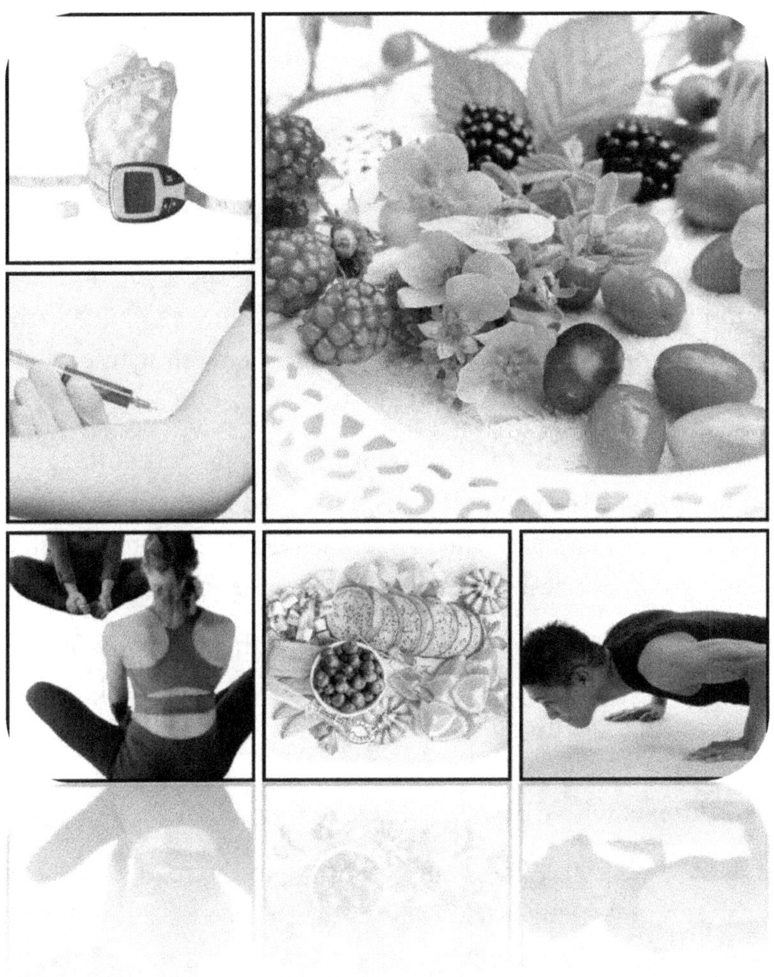

Remember that knowledge is power, and each step toward a healthy lifestyle leads to a brighter, diabetes-friendly future.

ACKNOWLEDGEMENT

I would like to express my deepest gratitude to everyone who contributed to the creation of this book, "Type 2 Diabetes For Beginners."

Firstly, I want to thank my family for their unwavering support and understanding during the countless hours spent researching, writing, and editing. Your encouragement has been my driving force.

A heartfelt appreciation goes to my friends and colleagues who provided valuable insights and feedback. Your perspectives and expertise have enriched the content of this book and made it more relatable to a wider audience.

I extend my sincere thanks to the healthcare professionals who shared their knowledge and experiences, helping to ensure the accuracy and credibility of the information presented. Your dedication to improving the lives of individuals with diabetes is truly commendable.

Lastly, I want to express my gratitude to the readers—those who are on their own journey with diabetes and those seeking to understand and support their loved ones. It is my hope that this book serves as a helpful companion in your pursuit of a healthier and more fulfilling life.

Thank you all for being an integral part of this project.

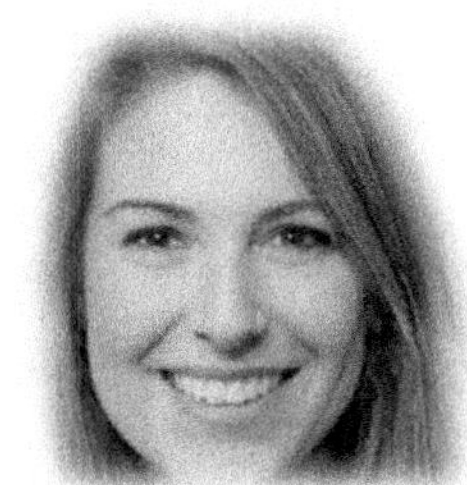

ABOUT THE AUTHOR

The Heart Behind the Words: Allison D. Dixon

In the vast realm of diabetic literature, Allison D. Dixon emerges not just as a seasoned dietician but as a compassionate storyteller with a profound connection to the narrative she weaves. Beyond the pages of nutritional advice and health strategies, there's a deeply personal tale that shapes the essence of this book

As the daughter of someone who embarked on the challenging journey of living with type 2 diabetes, Allison's perspective transcends the clinical realm. Witnessing her mother's struggles and triumphs ignited a fervent passion within her—an unwavering commitment to transforming the lives of those navigating the intricate landscape of diabetes.

This isn't just a guide; it's a testament to resilience, a chronicle of victories born from adversity.

In crafting this book, Allison carried not just her expertise as a dietician but the echoes of her mother's diabetes voyage. Every piece of advice, every empathetic word, and every practical strategy has been a companion on that journey. The book unfolds as a tapestry of shared experiences, making it a relatable and invaluable resource for those facing similar challenges.

But Allison's dedication doesn't end with these pages. She extends her support through a companion in the form of her "Type 2 Diabetes Cookbook," available on Amazon. A culinary journey that complements the wisdom shared in the book, providing a holistic approach to managing diabetes with flavorful and nourishing meals.

Join Allison on this heartfelt exploration of triumph over adversity. Let her words guide you, inspire you, and assure you that you're not alone in the challenges posed by diabetes. It's more than a book; it's a lifeline, cast out with love and understanding.

9 798884 614192